Alkaline Diet

I0090422

The Comprehensive Manual For Achieving Weight Loss,
Enhancing Vitality, And Restoring Optimal Health
Through The Application Of Alkaline Herbal Medicine To
Mitigate Degenerative Diseases

Malcolm Everett

TABLE OF CONTENT

An Exposition on the Alkaline Diet

Recently, there has been considerable enthusiasm regarding the alkaline diet. Its rapid rise in popularity prompts one to question the veracity of the surrounding acclaim.

It is a dietary regimen that enables individuals to substitute an acid-based diet with one entirely composed of alkaline properties.

The substitution of an alkaline-based diet with an acid-based diet has been deemed to be conducive to enhancing one's well-being and attaining a state of optimal physical health.

Conversely, proponents have asserted that substituting an acidic diet with this particular regimen can effectively deter the development of cancer, leading to a significant reduction in the individual's susceptibility to the disease. Individuals have been deeply impressed and captivated by this dietary regimen since its inception, vowing to exclusively adhere to it throughout their lifetime.

The rationale behind this belief is their perception that incorporating this dietary approach will enable them to attain their health objectives in a seemingly miraculous manner. Nevertheless, one might question the veracity of the purported benefits of this diet and whether it truly facilitates substantial personal improvement as it asserts. To ascertain the veracity of the matter, we cordially invite you to peruse this article, which will elucidate whether this option is deemed advantageous as per your discerning evaluation.

Familiarizing oneself with the principles of the alkaline diet:

Referred to as the alkaline diet, this nutritional approach is alternatively named the ash diet due to its absence of acidic components.

The rationale behind this dietary approach stems from the notion that when food is consumed, it undergoes a process of either being transformed into alkaline substances or substances possessing acidic properties.

The sustenance consumed undergoes a transformation within the body, resulting in a complete alteration as it is enzymatically disintegrated into smaller constituents. The metabolic process facilitates the modification of ingested food substances in order to facilitate optimal digestion.

This entire process is recognized as metabolism, wherein the food is transformed into either alkaline or acidic substances. The consumption of acidic food substances results in the generation of an acidic response within the stomach, which subsequently induces considerable discomfort and dissatisfaction. Consuming foods with acidic properties leads to the conversion of these substances into acids within the stomach, causing it to function in a manner similar to that of a furnace.

The residue produced by the food you consume may exhibit either acidic or alkaline properties.

When an individual consumes food with acidic properties, it is known to induce substantial acidic reactions within the body. This implies that the consumption of acidic food results in the body becoming acidic, whereas consuming food with alkaline properties causes the body to become alkaline.

The ingestion of food items containing acidic properties results in a diminished physiological state, rendering the individual more vulnerable and susceptible to various ailments and medical conditions.

Contrastingly, when an individual ingests food products containing alkaline properties, it is conceivable that a safeguarding barrier is formed around the body, assisting in the enhancement of overall health.

When one ingests food items with an alkaline composition, calcium and potassium are assimilated into the body, while the intake of acidic food items leads to an accumulation of sulfur within the body.

Numerous food items can be categorized as acidic, such as fish and meat, while others can be classified as alkaline, including vegetables and fruits.

Nevertheless, there are also food items with a neutral pH that do not lean towards acidity or alkalinity, such as fats and sugars. Therefore, it should be noted that the consumption of acidic food items may potentially lead to the manifestation of symptoms associated with acid reflux.

In contrast, including alkaline-rich foods in your daily dietary intake allows for the enhancement of the alkaline protective barrier surrounding your physical well-being.

The pH value:

The pH level of the dietary intake holds significance in the context of an alkaline-based diet.

Gaining an understanding of the significance of the pH value is of utmost importance, and it is imperative that one bears this in mind when embarking on the alkaline diet. The determination of pH value is a relatively straightforward process that effectively indicates the acidic or alkaline nature of a given consumable item.

Fundamentally, the pH value commences at 0 and culminates at 14. In the range of zero to seven, the substance is considered to have an acidic nature, whereas in the range of seven to ten, it is categorized as neutral. Nevertheless, once an individual surpasses a value of 10, the pH level veers towards alkalinity.

The pH level can be determined through a urine analysis, making it a straightforward process to ascertain the pH state of an individual's body.

"The influence of pH on the composition of your blood:

If one harbors the belief that the consumption of a specific type of sustenance can alter the pH level of one's bloodstream, it is an erroneous assumption.

The consumption of both acidic and alkaline food does not impact the pH equilibrium of the blood, rather, it predominantly influences the pH levels present in the urine. Therefore, it is important to note that the consumption of foods with acidic properties should not be presumed to impact the pH level of the blood, but rather it influences the pH value of the urine.

The Final Word

The alkaline diet undeniably bestows numerous favorable impacts upon the human body. Continuing a diet high in red meat over the course of a month will induce an acidic response in your stomach, creating an overall displeasing sensation.

Adopting the alkaline diet and consuming an abundance of vegetables and fruits effectively promotes the transformation of an unwell physique into a state of wellness.

Advantages of Adopting an Alkaline Diet

Curious about the advantages of alkaline diets? If that is the case, rest assured that there are countless individuals who share your desire to gain further knowledge about this nutritious dietary pattern, but they simply find themselves uncertain as to how to initiate their exploration. Hence, I am providing you with a comprehensive guide to aid your comprehension of the authentic nature of alkaline diets and the numerous benefits that can be derived from them.

This nutrition program is referred to by various names, such as the acid alkaline diet, the alkaline diet, and the alkaline ash diet. All of these terms denote identical fundamental principles, emphasizing the inclusion of fresh vegetables, fruits, whole grains, legumes, and nourishing oils.

What prompts the attraction towards alkaline diets?

Scientists acknowledge that the decomposition of substances in the body produces byproducts that can have either acidic or alkaline properties. Moreover, these byproducts possess the ability to impact the overall acid-alkaline equilibrium within the human organism. The optimal pH level of a healthy body leans towards alkalinity, but as we introduce increasingly acid-producing foods, the body grows more acidic. A state of acidity within the internal system leaves one vulnerable to various health issues.

A significant majority of the sustenance consumed by the average individual in contemporary times is extensively processed, characterized by elevated quantities of refined carbohydrates, unfavorable fats, sodium, and chemical additives that contribute to health-related issues. Sweet rolls, meats, and cream cheese elicit substantial acid production during the process of digestion and absorption. Processed food items contribute to the augmentation of acidic compounds. All of these acids are rapidly introduced into the bloodstream of the body, leading to complications as the body endeavors to maintain its regular alkaline pH balance.

According to experts in the field, it is recommended to maintain a pH level between 7.35 and 7.45. However, due to the considerably acidic nature of the typical American diet, it becomes challenging to uphold a healthy pH level, as indicated by authoritative figures in the alkaline diet community. These proponents hold the belief that by providing the body with the appropriate diet it was naturally designed for, one can achieve improved health and increased lifespan. Humans are naturally adapted to consume a dietary regimen consisting predominantly of fresh produce and unprocessed whole foods that have undergone minimal processing.

What are the advantages of adhering to alkaline diets?

As per the analysis of nutrition professionals, it is a diet characterized by acidity that is, to a certain extent, accountable for prevalent issues such as early onset of aging and persistent ailments. Health conditions such as arthritis and kidney stones are thought to be associated with diets known to produce excessive levels of acids within the body.

Transitioning to a low-acid diet is purported to have the potential to enhance vitality, diminish mucous production, alleviate irritability and anxiety symptoms, as well as potentially result in a decrease in both headaches and infections. Researchers are currently investigating assertions that an alkaline diet possesses the potential to mitigate bone density decline, muscle atrophy, urinary tract complications, and renal calculi.

If one were to inquire individuals adhering to these dietary regimens, they would attest to experiencing enhanced physical well-being, increased contentment, and heightened levels of energy when compared to individuals who embrace predominantly low-carbohydrate diets. Many individuals have discovered that their personal health problems have significantly diminished or completely resolved upon embracing alkaline diets. Shedding excess weight is also a prominent benefit for individuals who integrate whole foods into their lifestyles.

Maximizing the Benefits of an Alkaline Diet
Consulting a comprehensive list of specific food items can provide assistance, however, it is advisable to endeavor to consume a substantial quantity of fresh fruits and vegetables on a daily basis. Salads are consistently a favorable selection. Ensure adequate hydration by consuming generous

amounts of water, vegetable juices, or herbal infusions. Refrain from consuming processed foods, deep-fried items, chocolates, food products containing high levels of added sugars, and unhealthy junk foods. Rather than incorporating sugar or salt into the prepared dishes, consider utilizing nutritious and savory herbs and spices. Lastly, it is important to note that excessive cooking of food results in a significant loss of its nutritional content.

Consuming Alkaline-Rich Foods Can Alleviate Your Illness

Consuming foods with high alkaline levels can help maintain the body's pH balance and prevent acidification. If we consume alkaline-rich foods, the pH level of our body will naturally achieve equilibrium. Acidity occurs as a result of the consumption of foods that possess an acidic nature. Regrettably, it can be observed that Western diets tend to exhibit an overall acidic nature. This is the reason why it is imperative to balance acidity by incorporating foods with high alkalinity.

1.Eat fruits and vegetables. Fruits and vegetables serve as excellent sources of naturally occurring vitamins and minerals. Additionally, fruits and vegetables possess exceptional purifying properties for eliminating toxins from your body. It also effectively aids in promoting bowel movement, while simultaneously revitalizing the complexion and hair with their rich nutrient content.

2. Refrain from consuming alcohol and tobacco products. Smoking can lead to the development of lung cancer and other pulmonary diseases. Consumption of alcohol can lead to the development of liver cancer and other associated ailments. I experienced an instantaneous surge in vitality upon discontinuing these habits. In a matter of only a few weeks, I experienced a remarkable surge of energy and a renewed sense of youthfulness.

3. Exercised regularly. Please be advised that while a sedentary lifestyle may offer immediate comfort, embracing a healthy lifestyle will invariably contribute to an extended lifespan and an enhanced overall sense of happiness. If you find yourself lacking the availability to engage in daily exercise, it is advisable to maintain a consistent exercise routine during weekends or whenever you have leisure time throughout the week. Make an effort to participate in activities such as basketball or touch football. They offer an excellent comprehensive workout for the entire body.

Ensuring equilibrium of pH levels
The underlying principle of the pH miracle diet is the preservation of a harmonious pH balance. Consuming alkalizing foods is strongly recommended due to the slightly alkaline nature of the human body. When excessive consumption of acidic foods occurs, an imbalance is created within the digestive system, giving rise

to a multitude of complications such as weight gain, compromised immunity, fatigue, and diminished concentration. These issues can potentially lead to more severe health conditions.

Foods with acidic properties (to be avoided) and foods with alkalizing properties (to be emphasized) are the factors that contribute to the pH miracle diet. Consuming alkaline-rich foods assists in regulating the pH levels within your body, consequently promoting overall well-being. Numerous individuals lack comprehension regarding the definitions and interconnections of pH, alkali, acid, nutrition, and health.

The term 'basis' refers to a fundamental principle, and this specific term serves as the origin for the word 'basic'. The attributes of alkalinity and acidity are denoted as "Basic." The conditions in question are determined by the cellular composition of these food items. Therefore, the transition from an alkaline state to an acidic state cannot be achieved through external treatment. At their core, foods can be classified into alkaline or acidic categories.

From a chemical standpoint, alkaline and acidic substances can be regarded as antithetical. Whenever an acid reacts with a base, a salt is formed. "In a chemistry laboratory, these interactions are straightforward and simple." - In a laboratory setting dedicated to the study of chemistry, these interactions exhibit a characteristic quality of being transparent and uncomplicated. However, within our biological system, the interaction becomes more intricate due to the magnified scale at which the bases and acids come into contact.

In any event, researchers have formulated some generalizations regarding the impacts of alkaline substances and acids on our digestive system. In the human body, acidic foods give rise to acids. They reduce the pH levels of fluids such as saliva, lymph, and blood, rendering them more acidic. Consuming alkaline foods elevates the pH levels of these bodily fluids, rendering them alkaline in nature.

As a point of general reference, it should be noted that the typical pH range of human saliva is between 7.3 and 7.4. Nevertheless, it is worth mentioning that the majority of individuals tend to exhibit a lower pH value, indicating a higher degree of acidity. They are fatigued, exhausted, and their bodies crave equilibrium. Muscles are prone to exhaustion when subjected to the influence of acidic foods. Due to physical limitations, one is compelled to decelerate significantly as the body becomes incapable of achieving comparable outcomes as in the past.

When consuming acidic foods, oxidative stress occurs due to the formation of free radicals, leading to the process of aging. Minerals and vitamins are not readily assimilated. The digestive system experiences a disruption as beneficial microorganisms perish. Additionally, the proper functioning of the intestines is impaired due to the elevated acidity, resulting in diminished absorption of nutrients. Cells experience saturation with toxins that are incapable of being eliminated. The majority of the body's systems are incapable of functioning at their maximum capacity.

On the other hand, alkaline foods possess greater advantageous properties for one's overall well-being. Partaking in such dietary choices confers greater advantages. They possess antioxidative properties that can benefit the human body. The enhancement of assimilation at the cellular level contributes to the normalization of cellular performance. The provision of these food items contributes to a decrease in both yeast and parasitic proliferation. Consumption of alkaline foods promotes enhanced quality of sleep, rejuvenation of the skin, and alleviation of symptoms associated with colds, influenza, and headaches.

These food items also facilitate abundant physical energy.

The association with cancer represents a significant distinction between acidic and alkaline foods. In healthy tissues, alkalinity is observed, whereas cancerous tissues exhibit acidity. When oxygen reacts with an acidic fluid, it produces water as a result of the combination with hydrogen ions. Despite the corrective action of oxygen in neutralizing the acidity, the acid impedes the oxygen's access to the tissues. However, as oxygen gas enters an alkaline solution, it reacts with hydroxyl ions to generate one oxygen atom and one water molecule. The solitary oxygen molecule has the capacity to freely traverse to another cell and impart the beneficial properties of oxygen to the surrounding cells within the tissue. Cancer tissues enter a state of dormancy when the pH exceeds 7.4. Research has indicated that, when subjected to a pH level of 8.5, normal tissues thrive, whereas malignancies perish.

There are numerous advantages to adhering to an alkaline diet aside from its potential preventive effects against cancer. As you begin incorporating them into your physique

How does it Work

One notable aspect of the alkaline diet is its exemption from the necessity of monitoring caloric intake. The dietary regimen places emphasis on the quality of food consumed, rather than placing equal importance on the quantity of food consumed. Nevertheless, exercising prudence and refraining from excessive indulgence is advisable. Now is a suitable time to extensively explore the intricacies and rationales behind the dietary regimen. Only then will you gain a genuine comprehension of the immense advantages it offers you, as well as its remarkable effectiveness in facilitating weight loss and enhancing your overall well-being.

Allow us to revisit the pH scale in order to provide you with a comprehensive understanding of its critical significance. A pH level of 0 denotes complete acidity.

A pH level of 14 indicates a highly alkaline nature. The objective is to strive for a magnitude of 7, which would correspond to a state of neutrality. From a technical standpoint, it is essential for your stomach acid to maintain its acidity in order to adequately process and enzymatically break down the ingested food. The pH level of your stomach acid is approximately 3.5. Nevertheless, you are likely familiar with the sensation of burning or indigestion, which arises when excessive stomach acid reacts unfavorably as a result of consuming multiple acidic foods, thereby significantly lowering the pH level to a potentially harmful zero. You have consumed an excessive quantity of acidic food, thereby causing significant disruption to your digestive system.

Through the consumption of a nutritionally abundant diet consisting of alkaline foods, one can effectively maintain the acidity levels of their stomach at an optimal and easily controllable state. Consuming foods that produce acid can disrupt the functioning of your entire body. Our physical bodies are meticulously engineered mechanisms that necessitate meticulous supervision to operate optimally.

Continual consumption of food that elicits prolonged and heightened acid secretion in the body over an extended period may potentially lead to significant harm. The human body has the capacity to withstand occasional surges in acidity, but a persistent state of elevated acidity will have a detrimental impact on bodily functions. Your physical well-being will decline and you will experience an increase in body weight. Typically, those pounds tend to accumulate in the abdominal and gluteal regions. This is the location where your body will commence the storage of excess fat that it is unable to metabolize as a result of its disrupted and excessively strained physiological functioning.

Altering your dietary habits has the potential to significantly transform your life.

It is beneficial to have an awareness of your position on the pH scale in order to monitor your advancements. pH strips are available for purchase at a nearby pharmacy. In order to ascertain your pH level, it will be necessary to place one of the strips in the flow of your urine. It is advisable to utilize the urine produced during the second instance of urination within a 24-hour period. It is sufficient to conduct a pH test once within a span of 24 hours. This will aid in the determination of your dietary choices for the day. If your pH level is significantly lower than the optimal value of 7, it would be advisable to incorporate alkaline-dense foods, such as leafy green vegetables, into your diet to assist in raising your pH level.

The Broad Scope of the Alkaline Diet

The theory posits that the consumption of foods with high alkaline content results in the creation of an alkaline residue or ash. Currently, this ash is regarded as a mineral comprising essential elements such as calcium, iron, magnesium, copper, and zinc. These elements play a crucial role in upholding bodily homeostasis. Acidifying foods lead to a decrease in the levels of these crucial minerals, making our body more susceptible to various illnesses. Engaging in an alkaline diet helps safeguard the body and prevents such occurrences from taking place. In essence, it is crucial for our organism to uphold a pH level of 7.3. This implies that our body ought to maintain an alkaline state, a characteristic that should be mirrored in the composition of our dietary intake as well. The alkaline diet not only facilitates weight loss but also restores lost health and enhances longevity by preventing diseases.

Alluring, Refined, and Gourmet Recipes for Sustaining an Alkaline Diet

The alkaline diet encompasses the incorporation of higher quantities of vegetables into meals, the addition of a dash of lemon to water, the substitution of millet or quinoa for wheat, and the preference of olive oil over vegetable oil. Moreover, adhering to the diet involves the consumption of soups such as miso that align with its principles. Preparing a delectable midday meal consisting of a cucumber salad, which comprise of fresh tomatoes and cucumbers, along with a blend of balsamic vinegar, red wine, sea salt, minced garlic, fresh basil and oregano, and high-quality extra virgin olive oil. For the evening meal, a delectable dish can be prepared with vegetable pasta complemented by a rich tomato-pepper sauce. The essential ingredients include vegetable-based or spelled pasta, an assortment of both sun-dried and fresh tomatoes, a vibrant red bell pepper, a fresh zucc

Now, no meal can be considered complete without a dessert. Presented here are some guilt-free dessert options that are certain to satisfy your cravings. One such example is the classic apple pie, which can be prepared using ingredients such as ground raw walnuts, pitted dates soaked in alkaline water for 15 minutes, raw sunflower seeds, shredded apples, cinnamon, fresh apple juice, shredded coconut for garnishing, and either raisins or prunes. The dry ingredients, including those that have been soaked and drained, should be combined in a food processor to create the crust. To expedite the preparation of a dessert, one may assemble strawberries, blueberries, raspberries, blackberries, plain yogurt, and garnish with wheat germ and almonds to create a delectable dessert infused with various berries.

Discover the three uncomplicated alkalizing techniques that can be implemented immediately to swiftly attain enhanced vitality, vigor, and ideal body weight.

Efficient and Simplified Alkaline Diet Strategies

Following a diet that promotes alkalinity can serve as an effective means of enhancing your overall health and fostering a heightened sense of well-being. Although some individuals erroneously believe that adhering to an "alkaline diet" is intricate and arduous, it is, in fact, quite effortless to transition one's dietary habits from overly acidic to a nourishing and alkaline one. If you desire to partake in the myriad health advantages offered by an alkaline diet, there exist expeditious and effortless methods to achieve prompt outcomes. By transitioning to an alkaline diet, one can enjoy enhanced physical well-being, bolstered disease immunity, heightened energy levels, and an array of other advantageous outcomes.

Incorporate Alkaline Water into Your Dietary Regimen

Consuming an ample amount of water is a crucial component for maintaining optimal physical well-being. Therefore, it is worth considering the benefits of incorporating alkaline water into your daily routine. It is quite simple to produce homemade water by incorporating approximately half a teaspoon of baking soda into a gallon-sized container of water.

Agitate and evaluate using a pH strip, increasing the quantity of baking soda as necessary to attain a pH level ranging from 8.5 to 9. Alternatively, you may choose to utilize alkaline drops, tablets, or a jug filter, all of which can be easily obtained from commercial sources. You may also consider acquiring a water ionizer that can be effortlessly connected to your water source, ensuring unparalleled convenience. To enhance the taste and alkaline properties of your beverage, it is advisable to incorporate a squeeze of fresh lemon into your alkaline water prior to consumption. Additionally, this versatile ingredient can be utilized for the preparation of nutritious herbal and green teas, both of which serve as alkaline beverages.

Consume an abundant amount of salads. Incorporating salads comprising lettuce, spinach, and other verdant vegetables proves to be a beneficial inclusion as part of an alkaline diet. By incorporating a fresh salad comprising of vegetables into your lunch and dinner selections, you will not only promote your overall well-being but also enhance alkalinity within your body. Virtually all vegetables possess alkalizing properties, providing an ample array of options to ensure the enjoyable and captivating nature of your salads. Consider incorporating sliced cucumbers, snow peas, fresh green peas, and green pepper strips into your salad. Additional protein can be incorporated by including beans and other legumes.

Consume a reduced amount of sugar.

Refined sugar poses a significant detriment to an individual's well-being, particularly due to its propensity to promote an acidic physiological response. If you have developed a preference for the sweetness inherent in white sugar, I suggest reducing your consumption gradually to allow your taste receptors to acclimate. One may consider substituting white processed sugar with a small amount of raw sugar, maple sugar, or Stevia, all of which are viable options for sweetening that promote alkalinity. Nonetheless, refraining from substituting sugar with artificial sweeteners such as Equal, NutraSweet, or Sweet 'N Low is recommended, as they possess acidifying properties. Fortunately, as you begin to reduce the intake of sweeteners, you will notice a gradual inclination towards a less saccharine taste in your food.

Effortless Dietary Substitutions

It is quite straightforward to transition your diet from being highly acidifying to alkalizing by implementing a small number of straightforward food substitutions. In lieu of processed noodles and pasta, opt for whole grains such as millet, quinoa, and wild rice.

Substitute red meat in your dietary intake with fish, legumes, and other types of pulses as alternative sources of protein. Incorporate healthful fats into your meals, such as olive, flaxseed, or canola oil. In addition, it is advisable to consume a diet abundant in fresh fruits and vegetables as the majority of these possess alkalizing properties. In due course, you will experience an improvement in your well-being and enjoy the health advantages associated with adopting an alkaline diet.

The Hazards of the Alkaline Diet - Identifying Their Nature

Are you familiar with the concept of the Alkaline diet? Are you aware that it enjoys greater popularity even than the renowned South Beach Diet? This diet is widely regarded as one of the most fashionable regimens for achieving weight loss and fostering improved overall wellness. Nevertheless, are there any perils associated with adhering to an alkaline diet?

The alkaline diet has proven to be highly effective in facilitating the achievement of your optimal weight in accordance with your height and body type. This dietary regimen is designed to enhance your energy levels and promote an overall sense of well-being.

Nevertheless, despite adhering to an optimal dietary regimen, there are certain risks or perils involved. What are the key concerns one should address regarding the hazards associated with the alkaline diet?

The initial fact to be aware of is that it is not feasible to adhere to the alkaline diet in its entirety. It is advisable to incorporate acid-forming foods into your diet, and consuming meat is not inherently detrimental. The majority of individuals fail to comprehend the significance of balance in any dietary regimen. Without achieving a certain equilibrium, it is impossible to sustain a state of wellbeing.

It is important to note that this diet fails to address certain indispensable nutrients necessary for one's well-being. The alkaline diet lacks essential components such as fatty acids and nutrients like Omega 3 that are crucial for the proper functioning of your body. Once again, this is where the equilibrium arises. You have the option to incorporate items that do not adhere to the principles of the alkaline diet, as long as you counterbalance them with suitable alkaline foods and beverages.

One additional risk that you must comprehend is the impossibility of self-poisoning. It is somewhat peculiar to contemplate, but the consumption of bottled or tap water may contain certain toxins that are detrimental to one's physiological well-being. The plastic contains chemical substances that are detrimental to your health. The optimal course of action would be to utilize a filtration system and incorporate a portion of freshly cut lemon or lime to render your water alkaline.

Optimizing the Benefits of an Alkaline Diet: Effective Strategies

A proper alkaline diet entails maintaining a dietary composition where more than 80% of total food intake consists of alkalizing foods. This dietary regimen can be effectively adhered to by prioritizing the inclusion of substantial proportions of fruits and vegetables in one's daily intake, thereby attenuating ailments and decelerating the progression of aging. Although there are methods for determining the alkalizing foods, it may still pose a challenge to integrate the alkaline diet into our daily regimen. By adhering to specific guidelines of an alkaline diet, it is possible to effortlessly adhere to and integrate the diet into our lifelong daily routine.

Water and citrus juices are both considered alkaline foods. Therefore, it is advised to incorporate lemon juice into your glass of water as frequently as possible while following this diet. Lemon, despite being an acidic fruit, possesses alkalizing properties that benefit the body. It becomes laborious to prepare lemonade on a regular basis, particularly when sugar is required (unless one opts for stevia). In order to mitigate any discomfort while still reaping the benefits of the alkaline diet, incorporating a fresh lemon juice infusion into filtered water can effectively cater to the consumption of both mineral water and lemons.

One of the most straightforward approaches to adhering to an alkaline diet is to consume a substantial amount of fruits and vegetables. Regardless of the meal being consumed, it is recommended to incorporate a significant amount of vegetables and fruits into one's diet. Rather than consuming excessive amounts of bread, opting for a substantial portion of sautéed vegetables or a generous cabbage salad can be highly beneficial for maintaining an optimal pH level within your body. Thoroughly washed fruits can serve as a wholesome alternative to unappetizing and acidic evening snacks. Consider substituting a fresh apple or peach for a bag of potato chips. It is also beneficial to set aside one cup of alkalizing greens to be consumed throughout the day. Setting aside and consuming a cup of broccoli or kale throughout the day will guarantee the consumption of vegetables.

Wheat is acidic food. When following the alkaline diet, it is advisable to replace wheat with substitutes such as millet or quinoa. White bread should also be eliminated from consumption as it is considered to be acidic in nature. Opting for chicken instead of beef is preferable when one desires a delectable meat-based dish. Consider incorporating infrequent fish or lamb into your diet while striving to eliminate beef entirely from your meal choices. Simply substitute chicken for other types of meat in the various recipes, and you will be satisfactory.

Olive oil exhibits pronounced alkalizing properties and offers multiple advantageous effects. When adhering to an alkaline dietary regimen, it is recommended to abstain from vegetable and other oils, and instead prioritize the use of Olive oil. The intended purpose is to achieve radiant skin and luxurious hair as well. Incorporate a generous amount of leafy vegetables into your diet and introduce powdered greens as a supplement to virtually any meal. Miso is a food with a high alkaline content, and a simple broth can be prepared by adding a teaspoon of it to hot water. This soup can significantly augment the body's alkalinity levels.

The adoption of an alkaline diet as a long-term lifestyle choice is a convenient and sustainable alternative to engaging in crash diets. It effectively aids in maintaining an individual's weight within manageable levels, while simultaneously extending their lifespan. A life that is in good health brings value to everything.

1: Acid-forming Foods vs. Alkaline-forming Foods

Every type of food can be categorized as either alkaline-forming or acid-forming based on its impact on our physiological systems. A culinary item may exhibit sour and acidic qualities, much like lemon or lime, while still possessing an alkalizing impact on the body. This phenomenon may lead to confusion among individuals who anticipate that consumption of acidic foods would elicit an acidic response in the body.

The human body necessitates an equilibrium between acidity and alkalinity for optimal physical well-being and vitality. If the equilibrium is disrupted through the consumption of substantial quantities of acid-inducing foods, it will exert adverse consequences on the body, resulting in discomfort and fostering the onset of various ailments, including cancer. Presently, a considerable number of individuals consume a diet that comprises meat, wheat, dairy products, rice, pasta, pastries, and various other items that contribute to the acidification of the human body.

Degenerative conditions and other health ailments begin to manifest when the body turns excessively acidic due to the consumption of a greater quantity of acid-forming foods and a lesser amount of alkaline-forming foods, as opposed to the opposite scenario. Acidosis, or excessive acid levels within the body, stands as a primary etiological factor underlying numerous diseases. It is imperative to demonstrate vigilance in our dietary choices as they play a pivotal role in shaping the quality and duration of our lives. Indeed, the underlying cause of a majority of health conditions stems from acidosis; however, it is fortunately an avoidable occurrence. These medical conditions can be mitigated by the adoption of an alkaline diet.

Acidosis results in cellular acidification and oxygen deprivation. This creates a conducive environment for the proliferation of illnesses and diseases. The adoption of an alkaline diet can mitigate the acidity within the body induced by the consumption of a diet that promotes acidification. The adoption of an alkaline diet offers a substantial safeguard against afflictions such as cancer, cardiovascular diseases, stroke, kidney diseases, gallstones, anti-inflammatory diseases like osteoarthritis and rheumatoid arthritis, as well as obesity, along with various other medical conditions.

The Alkaline diet is alternatively referred to as the acid alkaline balance diet, the acid alkaline diet, or the cancer diet. The alkaline diet possesses the capacity to facilitate an optimal state of well-being, mitigate the risk of ailments, and potentially ameliorate medical conditions resultant from acidified body tissue.

All food items can be categorized into either acidogenic foods or alkalogenic foods. It is necessary for our bodies to obtain 20% of our dietary intake from foods that are acidic in nature, while the remaining 80% should consist of foods that are alkaline in nature. In order to uphold a natural balance between acidity and alkalinity for the sake of our well-being, it is imperative that we adhere to a ratio of 20 to 80 when it comes to acids and alkaline substances.

Regrettably, the dietary habits that a significant number of individuals presently adhere to are inclined towards a higher consumption of acid-forming foods, accompanied by a relative scarcity of alkaline-forming foods. Consequently, this has resulted in the prevalence of low-grade acidosis or chronic acidosis among a substantial portion of the population.

The circulatory system facilitates the distribution of nutrients and oxygen throughout the entire body, while simultaneously facilitating the elimination of carbon dioxide and other toxic waste products through various excretory organs such as the kidneys, lungs, and skin. Maintaining a proper pH balance in the bloodstream is vital for fostering overall bodily well-being, thereby emphasizing the importance of pH monitoring or embracing a nutritive regimen centered around alkaline-rich foods.

In order to maintain a state of well-being, it is imperative that the pH level of blood remains around 7.4, with a permissible deviation within the range of 7.37 to 7.43. In the event that the pH level of blood descends beneath 7.37 or ascends above 7.43, it provokes a state of decreased cellular activity in the body, leading to deteriorating tissue health and an inability to sustain ideal human well-being. Your physical resilience, capacity, and resistance to ailments and medical conditions are diminished.

It is imperative that you adhere to and embrace an alkaline diet, as doing so will effectively diminish the prevailing acidity in both your bloodstream and various bodily systems.

ALL ABOUT WATER

Why Drink Water?

The essential constituents of the human body, including blood, muscles, voice, and the brain, are composed predominantly of water. In order to regulate body temperature and facilitate the transportation of essential vitamins and minerals to the organs and tissues, it is imperative to ensure an adequate intake of water.

In addition, it aids in the delivery of oxygen to your cells, facilitates the removal of waste, and protects both your joints and internal organs. The insufficient intake of water results in dehydration. Indicators and manifestations of mild dehydration consist of a sensation of thirst, discomfort in muscles and joints, discomfort in the lower back, headaches, and irregularities in bowel movements.

The presence of a strong odor in your urine, accompanied by a yellow or amber hue, could indicate inadequate hydration.

Please take note that the consumption of dietary supplements that contain significant quantities of riboflavin, a B-vitamin, will result in the emission of noticeably altered urine coloration. Certain medications have the ability to alter the coloration of urine.

The excretion of water from the body occurs through processes such as urination, respiration, and perspiration, resulting in a higher loss of water during periods of physical exertion compared to periods of physical inactivity.

Substances such as diuretics, caffeine-containing beverages, certain pharmaceuticals, and alcoholic beverages have the potential to augment the amount of water excreted by the body. Lost bodily fluids must be replenished through the specific liquids present in the food you consume and the beverages you ingest.

What is the recommended amount of water that should be consumed? A minimum of 20% of the water required by your body is sourced from your diet. The remaining sources are derived from the beverages ingested.

A number of experts maintain that it is possible to estimate the quantity of water required by dividing one's weight in pounds and halving the resulting figure. Which specifies the recommended daily consumption in terms of ounces.

For instance, if you weigh 160 pounds, it is recommended to consume a minimum of 80 ounces of water or other hydrating fluids on a daily basis. Supplementary factors encompass the level of physical activity and the climatic conditions of your location. Our water vehicle loan calculator offers a means for you to determine the optimal daily water intake that suits your needs.

The consumption of water has emerged as the most optimal choice for rehydration owing to its cost-effectiveness and absence of caloric content or additional substances. Both tap and bottled water frequently undergo fluoridation in order to mitigate the occurrence of tooth decay.

Both sweetened carbonated beverages and non-alcoholic carbonated drinks are fortified with additional sugars, which contribute surplus energy from fat, without providing any supplementary nutrients or vitamins.

Sporting activities products contain minerals that aid in maintaining water balance, although it is important to be cautious of added sugars and calories that may not be desired.

Vegetable and fruit juices are typically a favorable choice owing to their rich mineral and vitamin content that caters to the essential needs of the body. Nevertheless, it is important to scrutinize the labeling, as certain plant-based fruit juices might contain excessive amounts of sodium. Beverages containing caffeine, like tea and coffee, also contribute to the tally. However, excessive intake of caffeine can induce a state of restlessness.

In recent years, there has been significant media coverage emphasizing the significance of consuming an ample amount of water and elucidating the adverse consequences of dehydration on the human body.

Water comprises roughly two thirds of the mass of a well-functioning human body, and it is this substantial water content that necessitates replenishment due to its loss through perspiration, urination, and respiration. Additionally, ongoing physiological processes within the body necessitate the presence of water in order to facilitate optimal functionality through chemical reactions.

The fundamental physiological processes within the human body are completely dependent on the presence of water. In the absence of an adequate quantity, the blood would be rendered incapable of transporting essential nutrients to the organs. Furthermore, water plays a pivotal role in facilitating the metabolic processes necessary for the body to effectively eliminate waste products.

Thirst serves as a critical indicator sent by the brain, signaling an urgent need for fluid replenishment. The cerebrum establishes communication with the renal system through the posterior pituitary gland, transmitting instructions regarding the desired volume of urine to be excreted and the appropriate quantity to be held in reserve.

Have you ever pondered the advantages of adopting alkaline diets? Rest assured that you are not alone in your desire to acquire additional knowledge about this nutritious dietary approach. However, many individuals struggle to determine the appropriate starting point for enhancing their understanding of the authentic fundamentals. Therefore, I am presenting you with a guide to assist you in acquiring knowledge pertaining to alkaline diets and the benefits that you can derive from them.

This nutritional program is referred to by various names, such as the acid alkaline diet, the alkaline diet, and the alkaline ash diet. All of these terms denote identical fundamental ideas emphasizing the inclusion of fresh vegetables, fruits, whole grains, legumes, and healthy oils.

What is the Reason Behind the Popularity of Alkaline Diets?

Scientists are aware of the fact that the decomposition of foods gives rise to byproducts that may be either acidic or alkaline. It has been recognized that these byproducts have the potential to affect the balance of acidity and alkalinity within the body. The optimal pH level of a healthy body is mildly alkaline, however, the introduction of acidic food items leads to an increase in the body's acidity. An individual's susceptibility to a wide range of health ailments increases with the presence of an imbalanced acidic physiological environment.

The majority of the foods consumed by individuals today are extensively processed, comprising substantial amounts of refined carbohydrates, unhealthy fats, sodium, and various chemicals that give rise to health concerns. Upon digestion and absorption, sweet rolls, meats, and cream cheese all generate a significant amount of acids. Processed food items contribute to the augmented presence of acidic compounds. All of these acids are rapidly released into the bloodstream of the body, thereby posing challenges as the body endeavors to maintain its typically alkaline pH equilibrium.

According to experts in the field, it is recommended that individuals maintain a pH level within the range of 7.35 to 7.45. However, achieving and sustaining a healthy pH level is challenging due to the prevalent consumption of highly acidic foods in the American diet, as noted by experts specializing in alkaline diets. These advocates contend that by providing the body with a diet that aligns with its inherent design, improved physical well-being and increased longevity can be accomplished. Humans are inherently suited for a dietary regimen comprising of fresh produce and other unprocessed whole foods with minimal alterations.

What are the Advantages of Alkaline Diets?

As per nutrition specialists, an acidic diet is deemed to be partially accountable for prevalent issues like premature aging and chronic ailments. Health conditions like arthritis and kidney stones are thought to be associated with diets that are known to produce an abundance of acids within the body.

Transitioning to a low-acid diet is purported to have the potential to enhance vitality, diminish mucus production, alleviate manifestations of restlessness and unease, and conceivably even result in a decreased incidence of headaches and infections. Scientists are currently investigating assertions that an alkaline diet possesses the ability to mitigate bone demineralization, muscle atrophy, urinary tract complications, and nephrolithiasis.

If one were to inquire individuals who abide by these dietary plans, they would indicate that they experience enhanced physical well-being, increased contentment, and heightened vitality compared to those adhering to other low carbohydrate diets. Many individuals have discovered that their personal health concerns have significantly diminished or been entirely eliminated upon embracing alkaline diets. Shedding excess body weight is also a significant benefit for individuals who adopt whole foods into their lifestyles.

Maximizing the Benefits of an Alkaline Diet

It is advantageous to consult a roster of particular food items, yet in general, one should strive to consume a copious amount of fresh fruits and vegetables on a daily basis. Salads consistently present themselves as a favorable option. Ensure adequate hydration by consuming ample amounts of water, vegetable juice, or herbal teas. Refrain from consuming processed foods, fried foods, chocolates, food items containing added sugars, and junk foods. Rather than incorporating sugar or salt into the dishes you prepare, consider utilizing nutritious and flavorful herbs and spices.

The food consumed in modern times significantly diverges from the dietary habits of our ancestors and bears little resemblance to the customary fare we have grown accustomed to today. As eloquently expressed, "Our dietary choices play a significant role in shaping who we are. In light of technological progress, the quality of the foods we consume can have a profound impact on our overall well-being." A glimpse inside the grocery store will astound you with numerous aisles filled with an extensive range of processed food items and animal-derived products. With the current widespread accessibility of fast foods, locating them in our local communities presents no challenge.

Partial responsibility can be attributed to fad diets for their role in introducing novel eating patterns, including but not limited to high-protein diets. In recent times, there has been a notable surge in the ingestion of animal-derived food products and processed food items, as an increasing number of individuals have been excluding the regular intake of fruits and vegetables from their dietary choices.

It is not surprising that in contemporary times, a significant number of individuals are afflicted by a multitude of ailments and allergies, encompassing various conditions such as bone disorders, cardiovascular issues, and numerous other illnesses. Several health professionals associate these diseases with the type of diet we consume. Certain types of food have the ability to disturb the equilibrium within our bodies, which gives rise to health issues during such instances. If we do not alter our dietary patterns, it is improbable that the prevention of ailments and restoration of well-being can be attained.

Low pH Levels: Exploring the Consequences of Acidity within the Human Body

Each and every bodily fluid possesses a unique and optimal pH range, indicative of good health. As an illustration, the pH of oxygen-rich arterial blood is rigorously maintained within a marginally alkaline pH spectrum of 7.35 to 7.45. Optimal cellular and tissue functioning, as well as overall health, necessitate the presence of an alkaline milieu in the body. The overall state of the body's health relies on its ability to uphold a natural state of balance, known as homeostasis, which diligently regulates the pH level.

The pH levels of saliva and urine can be indicative of an individual's dietary choices. Throughout the course of the day, the pH levels of saliva and urine may fluctuate within a range of acidity, measuring 5.5, to alkalinity, measuring 8. With the exclusion of pure water, all remaining edibles undergo either acid or alkaline formation upon consumption. The acidic or alkaline nature of any food is determined by the compounds or residues that are generated as a result of its metabolic processes within the human body. The pH level of a food is not considered to be equivalent to its pH value when not within the confines of your body.

Consequently, fruits and vegetables that contain substantial amounts of potassium tend to possess strong alkalizing properties, as potassium exerts a significant influence on alkalinity. Conversely, high-protein foods tend to have an acidifying effect as they contain sulfur and phosphorus, which result in the production of acidic residues during metabolism. All categories of alcoholic beverages, caffeinated beverages such as coffee, as well as carbonated beverages are recognized as acid-forming within the human body. Similarly, processed and sugary food items, dairy products, meat, poultry, as well as fish and seafood, exhibit an acidic nature.

Alkaline-predominant foods will contribute to maintaining homeostasis and safeguarding the crucial reserves of alkalinity within the body. In order to preserve homeostasis in the body following the intake of foods that promote acidity, it becomes necessary to counterbalance the acidic remnants with alkaline substances and subsequently eliminate them from the body. Over a period of time, the consumption of acidifying processed, sugary, and high-protein foods will lead to excessive strain on the body's buffering mechanisms, primarily due to the fact that the body has a finite daily capacity for the elimination of acid. When the body becomes unable to adequately fulfill the high demands associated with waste removal, it will proceed to retain the surplus acid in tissues for subsequent elimination.

The accumulation of acidic substances in bodily tissues can establish conditions conducive to the onset of various ailments and disorders, such as persistent exhaustion, diminished bone density, and malignant neoplasms. Metabolic acidosis is the term used to describe the accumulation of acid within the body.

Metabolic acidosis may arise as a consequence of excessive acid production in the body or due to compromised renal capacity to adequately eliminate acid from the body. There exist alternative types of acidosis that may not be directly correlated with dietary factors. Lactic acidosis is a form of metabolic acidosis resulting from the accumulation of lactic acids in the body. It arises due to hepatic failure, oncological conditions, hypoglycemia, profound anemia, or excessive alcohol consumption.

Hyperchloremic acidosis can also be described as an acid-base disturbance resulting from the depletion of sodium bicarbonate, which is an alkalizing agent, in the event of acute diarrhea. The prevailing type of acidosis observed in the general populace is chronic low-grade metabolic acidosis, which arises as a result of the conventional dietary practices characterized by a significant intake of foods that promote acid formation.

Chronic metabolic acidosis hampers cellular functioning by compromising electron transport, resulting in elevated energy expenditure and diminished energy generation. The disruption of electron transport within the cells lays the groundwork for persistent exhaustion and compromised immune function. Moreover, acidosis has the potential to enhance the generation of harmful free radicals within cells and hinder the functioning of antioxidants, thereby giving rise to persistent inflammation or even cancer. Research has demonstrated that the decline in alkaline reserves has a direct correlation with the development of osteoporosis.

The elevation of acidity levels in the bloodstream, tissues, and cells of the body, which occurs as a direct result of consuming snacks, fast foods, processed foods, sweets, products containing yeast, and various other foods that promote acidity, could potentially disrupt the efficient generation of energy and exacerbate weight gain. The inherent response of the human body to an excessive level of acidity involves the sequestration of acidic waste within adipocytes and adipose tissue, thereby safeguarding vital organs against the detrimental effects of heightened acidity. The condition known as acidosis, which is characterized by excessive acidification of body fluids or cells, is a contributing factor to obesity and is implicated in numerous ailments resulting from the impairment of cellular activities and functions. In an effort to safeguard against acidosis and potential harm, the body will form new adipocytes with the objective of containing the surplus acid within its system.

If one consistently encounters sensations of fatigue, headaches, and frequently exhibits symptoms akin to common colds and the flu, it is plausible that an individual may be harboring an elevated level of acidity within the body.

71

The repercussions of acidosis on the body not only exacerbate typical ailments, but also have the potential to induce additional conditions.

Some of the conditions associated with elevated levels of acidity in the body include but are not limited to depression, gastric ulcers, dry skin, acne, and obesity. In addition to the aforementioned conditions, other significant and grave illnesses, including but not limited to joint disorders, osteoporosis, bronchitis, recurrent infections, and cardiac ailments.

Further exploring, unraveling the enigma surrounding the alkaline diet

In simpler terms, pH serves as an indicator of the acidity level present in a given substance. The complete pH scale encompasses a range of values from 1 to 14. Substances exhibiting a pH value below 6 are referred to as acidic. A pH value of 7 indicates a state of neutrality, whereas any value exceeding this threshold is classified as alkaline. As the pH values decrease, the acidity levels increase. As the value increases, the substance exhibits a higher alkalinity.

The pH value of the food we consume also shows a range of variation; certain substances are abundant in acids, while others tend to be more alkaline in nature. A clear distinction between a purely alkaline diet and a non-alkaline diet is lacking, aside from the practice of recognizing and avoiding items with low pH levels. Items such as lemons, oranges, meat, dairy products, and processed food exhibit acidic properties.

Testing Your pH level

After making the decision to adopt the alkaline diet, it is essential to gradually strategize and implement incremental modifications in your lifestyle. It is not advisable to hastily adopt the initial diet plan encountered, as individual differences exist. In order to maximize the benefits of this diet plan, it is essential to gain insight into your pH level prior to proceeding. In order to accomplish this, it is imperative to evaluate your acid levels and determine their respective placement on the pH scale.

It is quite straightforward to conduct tests to determine the acidic levels in your body. It is necessary for you to obtain pH test paper. This study examines the acidity and alkalinity levels of any fluid originating from the human body. You have the option to utilize either urine or saliva as means for assessing your acidic levels. Nevertheless, it is strongly advised that you conduct the test using the initial urine sample obtained in the morning following a minimum of 6 hours of undisturbed rest. To conduct the examination, simply acquire a strip of paper and immerse it within a vessel containing accumulated urine or directly expose the paper to your urine. If you experience any discomfort in voiding urine, an alternative option would be to expectorate onto the paper immediately upon awakening in the morning.

Upon purchase of the pH paper test, a complimentary color chart will be provided to assist you in determining the acidity level of your body. The spectrum of hues spans from yellow to blue, accompanied by numerical markings. As previously stated, individuals with a pH value below seven are inclined towards acidity, while those with a pH value above seven are indicative of a state of wellness.

It is advisable to acquire pH test paper and employ it periodically. The rational behind this is that, by adhering to the diet plan, you will systematically assess your progress at regular intervals. These findings will assist in maintaining elevated levels of motivation.

The alkaline diet, alternatively referred to as the acid-alkaline diet,

Alkaline diet

The prevalence of current low carbohydrate and high protein diets represents a potential jeopardy to one's overall well-being. To maintain a physically fit physique, it is essential to abstain from following such dietary regimens. These diets not only lead to profound fatigue, but they also prove to be detrimental when it comes to weight control. Opting for an alkaline diet regimen is the sole approach to attain optimal well-being and effectively eliminate surplus weight.

The adoption of an alkaline diet necessitates adhering to a lifestyle paradigm completely divergent from that of high protein, low carbohydrate dietary regimens. The individual adhering to the high protein dietary regimen experiences feelings of fatigue and exhaustion. This program is designed for individuals who live a sedentary lifestyle and aim to reduce their body mass. Nevertheless, the lost weight promptly returns once the diet is discontinued. This does not hold true for alkaline diets. The dietary plans can be seamlessly integrated into an individual's lifestyle, and within a short span of time, noticeable results become apparent. To ensure efficacy, it is necessary for individuals adhering to the diet to consume approximately 80% of alkalizing foods, so as to maintain a body pH of 7.4, which is optimal for alkalinity. In general, diets high in protein tend to induce an acidic pH level in the body, deviating from its natural inclination towards alkalinity. When the body's pH level becomes acidic, it becomes susceptible to illnesses and experiences a depletion of energy. An acidic pH is also associated with the rapid deterioration of human body cells. This results in a diminished lifespan. It is imperative to avoid engaging in crash diets and explore the pursuit of health and vitality through the adoption of alkaline diets instead.

Alkaline diet plans facilitate the maintenance of the body's alkaline pH balance. The myriad bodily functions operate harmoniously, ensuring the maintenance of a robust immune system. To clarify, alkaline diet plans seem to aid in the prevention of diseases, whereas high protein diets seem to increase susceptibility to them.

Alkaline diets are suitable for individuals of all demographics. It is imperative for each individual to refrain from subjecting their bodies to harmful practices and instead prioritize the cultivation of a healthy and prolonged existence through the incorporation of alkaline diets into our daily routines.

Acid-alkaline diet

If you are familiar with the Atkins diet, it can be understood that the acid alkaline diet is its complete opposite. The Atkins diet regimen is characterized by its emphasis on a high protein and high fat intake, while significantly limiting carbohydrate consumption. A diet regimen referred to as an acid alkali, alkaline ash diet plan, alkaline acid diet, or simply the alkaline diet, effectively maintains a properly balanced pH level in the body, thus providing protection against various health ailments.

The underlying principle of an acid alkaline diet plan is predicated on the necessity of maintaining a body pH level of 7.4. This moderately alkaline pH level contributes to the optimal functioning of vital organs and enhances mineral retention within the body. When the pH level shifts towards acidity, challenges arise. An elevated pH level is known to impact nearly all bodily components in some form or the other. Given that our physiological makeup ought to be inclined towards alkalinity, it is imperative that this reflects in our dietary practices. Alkalizing foods necessitate a greater intake in comparison to acidifying foods. This would indicate a greater emphasis on consumption of vegetables and fruits, while significantly reducing the consumption of meat and oils. When the alkaline mineral levels in the body, specifically magnesium, calcium, and potassium, decrease, its overall health will decline, leading to degeneration and a decrease in its defense mechanisms. Adherence to an alkaline diet prevents such an occurrence. A diet regimen characterized by the presence of corrosive alkaline substances or alkaline debris consists of 80% alkalizing foods and 20% acidic foods.

The potential for experiencing pressure and a decreased level of vitality may be alleviated through the consumption of an alkaline diet that helps balance acidity. Those individuals who suffer from chronic viral fevers or nasal congestions can lead a more improved quality of life if they adhere to an alkaline diet.

An enhanced emphasis on the consumption of vegetables is suggested in an alkaline residue diet regimen. It is imperative to extract the essence of lemons and incorporate it into beverage preparations. Millet or quinoa is favored over wheat, olive oil over oil and soups like miso are extremely advantageous for following an alkaline debris diet plan.

By adhering to an acid alkaline diet, one can reinstate their lost state of health and vitality. Numerous chronic conditions can be both prevented and managed. This is a relatively uncomplicated dietary program, intended to promote an extended and more robust lifespan.

Raw Buckwheat Porridge for an Alkaline Diet

INGREDIENTS:

- 1 banana
- 2 ½ blueberries
- 2tsp acai berry powder
- 3tbsp water

- 3 oz. raw buckwheat kernels
- 1 ½ gluten free porridge oats
- 2 tsp. golden linseeds
- 4 dates
- Water to cover

INSTRUCTIONS:

• Combine the buckwheat kernels, oats, linseeds, and dates. • Blend the buckwheat kernels, oats, linseeds, and dates. • Integrate the buckwheat kernels, oats, linseeds, and dates. • Meld together the buckwheat kernels, oats, linseeds, and dates. • Merge the buckwheat kernels, oats, linseeds, and dates. • Unify the buckwheat kernels, oats, linseeds, and dates.

• Immerse in water and allow it to soak for a duration of one hour.

• After the buckwheat has become tender, discard the water.

• Transfer the ingredients to a high-speed blender, including the banana, and pulse until a consistency resembling porridge is achieved.

•Combine the blueberries, water, and acai berry powder in a saucepan and gently heat until the berries disintegrate, resulting in a dense sauce.

•Transfer the porridge into individual bowls and garnish it with a generous serving of the blueberry sauce.

The Long-Term Health Advantages of Incorporating an Alkaline Diet

Upon your decision to adopt the Alkaline diet and embark on a journey towards a wholesome lifestyle, or in the event that you are facing any ailments, this endeavor aims to promote your path to restoration. Although there may be individuals who yearn for the inclusion of meat in their diet, it is possible to achieve equilibrium by adhering to the 80/20 principle. This principle entails consuming 80 percent Alkaline foods and 20 percent Acidic foods, thereby ensuring a harmonious blend and sufficient intake of Alkaline foods to maintain an optimal and healthy pH level.

Since the Alkaline Diet serves as a protracted approach aimed at restoring and maintaining the body's equilibrium, it occasions numerous internal transformations that may elude our direct observation. Nevertheless, the advantageous outcomes of these alterations still accrue to us. As the duration of your adherence to the diet increases, the benefits you can obtain will grow correspondingly and significantly. Extensive research has been carried out, yielding findings that indicate diseases and illnesses are incapable of thriving in a physiological environment characterized by alkalinity. This theory has already demonstrated its efficacy and holds immense potential for further accomplishments. Individuals have reported improvements in their skin conditions, weight reduction, and even alleviation of symptoms associated with depression after incorporating greens into their diets, whether by consumption or through juicing, as some prefer in contemporary times. Certain individuals who previously suffered from persistent hay fever have ceased their reliance on medication, while others articulate that their diabetes has been effectively reversed and they have experienced significant improvement in peripheral circulation with minimal swelling. Furthermore, it is noteworthy that certain individuals have presented significant testimonials affirming the reversal of cancer and heart disease symptoms, without experiencing any adverse effects.

Previous research has demonstrated that extended timeframes can lead to enhancements in individuals suffering from back pain and muscular atrophy. These health conditions are presumed to be associated with the phenomenon that, once the human body acquires an acidic state, the bones progressively lose essential nutrients.

Similar to the majority of dietary plans, there may be a few transient consequences experienced within the initial days, such as the occurrence of headaches, fatigue, and slight lightheadedness. However, it is important to note that these are common and not cause for concern, as they will swiftly subside. Subsequently, following the detoxification of your body, you will begin to experience the advantages, including heightened energy levels, enhanced skin condition, and an improved mood. You will perceive a discernible enhancement in both your emotional state and your level of focus.

The Alkaline diet can be regarded as a highly commendable dietary approach, distinct from many passing trends, as it represents a return to the dietary practices of earlier times. In those days, before the advent of industrialized food processing and the use of harmful insecticides and pesticides that are prevalent in today's modern world, people consumed food in a manner that was more aligned with natural and healthful principles. Consuming a well-rounded diet comprising fruits and vegetables was inherently ingrained in our daily lifestyle. Regrettably, it is only in recent times that our food crop processing has undergone industrialization, and we are now witnessing its consequences on a daily basis.

On a daily basis, we are inundated with accounts of individuals succumbing to illness, experiencing weight gain, and receiving diagnoses for various ailments. A significant portion of these issues can be attributed to the dietary choices made by the average individual, with salt and chronic acidity emerging as prominent contributors in this regard. Once an individual adopts the Alkaline diet, the consumption of processed salt will be significantly diminished. This intervention is designed to enhance arterial health, facilitating the smooth circulation of blood throughout the body. This, in turn, alleviates stress on the heart and fosters improved blood flow. The enhanced circulation resulting from this phenomenon facilitates the effective transportation of oxygen throughout the body, including the brain. Consequently, individuals afflicted with diabetes, a condition frequently associated with impaired blood flow in extremities, will witness notable enhancements.

Children are an additional demographic that experiences the repercussions of acidosis. It has been observed that they may suffer from a deficiency in growth hormone, but this issue can be addressed by elevating the levels of bicarbonate and potassium citrate. The implementation of the 80/20 concept is essential as it enables the body to effectively stimulate the production of the growth hormone, thereby facilitating natural growth and safeguarding against various illnesses and diseases.

Additionally, research has revealed that postmenopausal women experience restricted growth hormone development. Therefore, through elevating the potassium bicarbonate levels in these women, it can effectively result in enhanced quality of life, enhanced body posture, as well as improvements in memory.

If you do not have any significant health issues, and you opt to adopt the Alkaline diet with the sole purpose of promoting a sense of well-being, achieving weight loss, and restoring your bodily equilibrium, you will observe a noticeable surge in energy levels throughout the duration of the day. It has been suggested that one may experience improved sleep patterns and heightened sexual satisfaction. You will experience enhanced skin condition, your hair will exhibit a stronger state of health, and your emotional state will be uplifted. It is challenging to determine with certainty the potential long-term effects of the Alkaline diet on individuals with significant medical conditions, given that their bodies may require a more substantial effort to restore balance due to the severity of such ailments. It is anticipated that enhancements will be expeditiously witnessed, and upon successfully surmounting your physical discomfort, you shall experience an amelioration in various aspects such as skin condition and quality of sleep.

Like many transient diets, the Alkaline diet is not without its disadvantages when followed over an extended period. However, it should be noted that this dietary approach represents more of a lifestyle choice, capable of conforming to the 80/20 principle, which entails limiting the consumption of acidic foods to a minimum. By adhering to this principle, one can ensure the appropriate intake of essential fatty acids necessary for optimal bodily functioning. In accordance with this objective, there are no significant records that indicate the unsuitability of the Alkaline diet for extended durations. Regard it as a transformation of your lifestyle, and be aware that attaining this goal is indeed possible by adhering to the principle of the 80/20 rule. You have the opportunity to attain a remarkable appearance and demeanor while occasionally indulging yourself. It undeniably represents a sustainable option, facilitating an enhanced quality of life through improved nutritional intake.

PH And The Body

As previously stated, pH is utilized as a means of assessing the alkalinity or acidity of a given solution. In the event that the pH is low, there will be a correspondingly high concentration of hydrogen ions, and conversely, in instances where the pH is high, a low concentration of hydrogen ions can be expected. If the optimal pH level within any of the body's systems deviates either towards acidity or alkalinity, it can give rise to a plethora of issues within the body.

The maintenance of an optimal pH level in the bloodstream is of paramount significance for ensuring the proper functioning of physiological processes within the body. The typical pH level observed in the circulatory system is approximately 7.35. The human body exerts significant effort to maintain the stability of that numerical value. In the event of a pH level deviation exceeding a range of approximately one to two units in the bloodstream, the entire electrical system within the physiological framework would cease to operate, inevitably resulting in the demise of the individual. It is of utmost importance to maintain a stable pH level in the bloodstream.

The erythrocytes transport oxygen to the different cellular entities within the organism. As red blood cells traverse the circulatory system, they will ultimately come across capillaries, diminutive branches that diverge from the primary pathways of blood veins and penetrate the anatomical regions inaccessible to blood veins. These capillaries possess dimensions so minuscule that the norm for red blood cells is to undertake their traversal in single-cell succession, as opposed to the accustomed method of traveling in larger aggregates. As the red blood cells are required to disperse from one another and function autonomously, they are enveloped by a substance that possesses an inherent negative charge. This results in cellular separation due to their inability to adhere to each other.

It is crucial to be cognizant of the factors capable of significantly disrupting the pH level of blood to the extent that bodily functions may cease entirely. The principal instigator in this scenario is the generation of acidity within the physiological system. The acidic nature inhibits the mobility of red blood cells by gradually eroding their membrane, which is the very membrane responsible for preventing their agglutination. Furthermore, in the absence of this protective coating, the cells tend to adhere to one another readily. Thus, rather than circulating unhindered within the bloodstream, these substances tend to aggregate into discrete clusters dispersed throughout the entire body. This can pose a significant challenge to the smooth passage of red blood cells through the blood vessels. The red blood cells are unable to traverse the minuscule capillaries. Consequently, there is a significantly reduced supply of oxygen being delivered to the body's cells.

Moreover, the process engenders a self-perpetuating cycle of negativity. As the acid gradually erodes the red blood cells, they will ultimately succumb to their demise. Once the red blood cells reach the end of their lifespan, they excrete an increased amount of acid that subsequently corrodes additional red blood cells. To summarize, the sole acid present in the human body that contributes to its well-being is the acid secreted within the stomach to facilitate the process of digestion. Thus, with the elevation of acid levels in the body, accompanied by the subsequent death of red blood cells resulting in diminished oxygen transportation to the cells, a significant physiological imbalance ensues. The individual experiences a significant decline in their level of energy.

The blood's pH level is distinct from that of other regions within the body. Every region of the body maintains its own distinct pH level, and the body exerts considerable effort to preserve optimal pH levels across all bodily regions. The pH level of the saliva varies from that of the upper region of the stomach. The pH level of the lower region of the stomach differs from that of the upper portion. The gastrointestinal system possesses an independent pH level. It is imperative to maintain these levels in order to uphold the proper functioning of their respective functions. The body ensures the maintenance of distinct pH levels through the utilization of three distinct mechanisms: renal control, respiratory control, and the buffer systems.

A component of the buffer system comprises proteins. These proteins will exhibit either donor or acceptor properties, depending on the prevailing acidity or alkalinity of the system. Buffers play a crucial role in maintaining system stability, particularly during instances when equilibrium can rapidly be disrupted, such as periods of heightened strain or intense physical exertion.

The regulation of the respiratory system holds particular significance. When individuals respire, they inhale oxygen which is subsequently assimilated into the organism, while carbon dioxide (CO_2) is expelled from the body through exhalation. Carbon dioxide (CO_2) is a byproduct generated by cellular activities. The red blood cells serve the essential function of facilitating the transportation of oxygen into the body's cells and aiding in the removal of carbon dioxide, which is then exhaled via the respiratory system. When individuals voluntarily cease breathing, there is an elevation in the carbon dioxide (CO_2) concentration within the bloodstream, resulting in a resultant decrease in the blood's pH level, which may precipitate a loss of consciousness. Maintaining optimal blood pH level requires careful regulation of breathing patterns and effective control over the respiratory process.

Understanding Acid-Alkaline Balance

The state of well-being is indeed the result of the harmonious coordination of all physiological mechanisms within the human body. The cells comprising our physiological framework are incredibly interconnected, such that any enhancement in the equilibrium of a particular system yields a corresponding amelioration in the equilibrium and robustness of all other organ systems.

As an illustration, enhancing cardiovascular well-being yields improvements in digestive functionality. Enhancing the functionality of the nervous system will lead to enhancements in the lymphatic system, and of utmost significance, when one enhances the acid/alkaline equilibrium of the body, simultaneous enhancements occur in all other bodily systems.

The pursuit of equilibrium initiates within our circulatory system, just as does the process of mending wounds, diminishing inflammation, promoting lipid combustion, fortifying skeletal structure (reversing osteoporosis), and augmenting vigor and vitality.

For proper functioning, it is essential that the blood and other bodily fluids maintain an extremely precise acid/alkaline balance, as indicated by the pH factor (potential hydrogen). The pH scale spans from 0 to 14, encompassing extreme acidity to extreme alkalinity. Anything with a pH value below 7.0 can be classified as acidic, whereas anything above 7 is considered alkaline. It is important to note that there is a tenfold difference between each number when testing the pH. To provide an illustration, a pH value of 5.0 denotes that the solution is tenfold more acidic compared to a pH value of 6.0.

The pH of blood does not readily undergo changes. The pH level of our blood falls within the range of 7.25-7.45. Should the pH deviate outside this specified range, it would disrupt the proper functioning of the body.

A significant quantity of energy is utilized to uphold pH levels, simultaneously depleting the body's alkaline mineral reserves, resulting in deficiencies and health disorders.

By ensuring optimal pH levels are consistently upheld, the process of injury healing is accelerated, and health complications exhibit improved rates of recovery. This is attributed to enhanced oxygenation of the body, which facilitates detoxification and self-healing mechanisms.

When cells are activated through this mechanism, it leads to the development of a robust immune response against diseases and a notably decreased predisposition to cancer.

The most effective approach to maintaining optimal pH levels and vitality entails monitoring our dietary and beverage choices, as well as managing our responses to stress. When adhering to the diet, embracing an 80/20 ratio of alkaline-forming foods to acid-forming foods will likely enable you to derive all the advantages associated with achieving bodily equilibrium.

Please peruse the subsequent lists to ascertain the effects of various foods and identify potential means of augmenting your intake of alkaline-forming foods. Please be advised that it is crucial to ensure that the foods used are of an organic nature, as all pesticides have highly acidic properties.

FOODS THAT HAVE AN ALKALINE EFFECT ON THE BODY:

Dairy products: acidophilus, whey, kefir/yogurt

FRUITS: apples, apricots, avocados, bananas, berries, cantaloupes, cherries, currants, dates, figs, grapes, grapefruits, guavas, lemons, limes, mangoes, melons, nectarines, oranges, papayas, passion fruits, peaches, pears, persimmons, pineapples, raisins, strawberries, tangerines. Alternative phrasing: The selection of fruits available includes apples, apricots, avocados, bananas, berries, cantaloupes, cherries, currants, dates, figs, grapes, grapefruits, guavas, lemons, limes, mangoes, melons, nectarines, oranges, papayas, passion fruits, peaches, pears, persimmons, pineapples, raisins, strawberries, and tangerines.

VEGETABLES: bamboo shoots, green beans, lima beans, string beans, sprouts, beets, broccoli, cabbage, carrots, celery, cauliflower, chard, chicory, chives, collard greens, cucumber, dandelion greens, dill, dulse, eggplant, endive, escarole, kale, garlic, leeks, legumes, lettuce, okra, onions, parsley, parsnips, sweet potato/yam, bell peppers, white potatoes, pumpkin, radish, rutabaga, turnips, watercress.

MEAT: There is no alkalinity present in meat.

NUTS: comprised of almonds, chestnuts, and coconuts.

MISCELLANEOUS: ginger, honey, kelp, alfalfa, clover, mint, sage, green tea, quinoa, flaxseed, pumpkin seeds, all types of seaweed and sea vegetables.

Essential minerals present: calcium, magnesium, potassium, manganese

ACIDIFYING FOODS

Cereal Grains: inclusive of all refined flour products, buckwheat, wheat, corn, barley, oats, rye

DAIRY PRODUCTS: butter, eggs, cheese, cottage cheese, cream, ice cream, custards, milk

Varieties of fruits to consider include preserves, cranberries, pomegranates, and olives.

VEGETABLES: artichokes, asparagus, garbanzo beans

MEAT: All

NUTS: Including but not limited to peanuts, pistachios, walnuts, and macadamia nuts.

Alcoholic beverages, brine, coffee, cocoa/chocolate, confectionery, numerous dressings (due to the presence of vinegar), pharmaceutical drugs, preserves, mayonnaise, certain seasonings, carbonated beverages, sleep deprivation, stress, anxiety.

ASSESSING YOUR ACID-BASE BALANCE

In the realm of bodily health, regular and slight variances in the internal pH levels are customary, necessitating the utilization of various methods to evaluate and discern one's pH level. This course of action is integral in obtaining comprehensive insights into one's overall well-being.

Similar to a swimming pool, the human body is predominantly composed of water. Consequently, it is imperative to maintain a harmonious pH level. The most effective approach to achieving this equilibrium is by assessing the pH status within one's system.

Through the vigilant observation of your pH level over a prolonged duration, you will be able to discern recurring tendencies towards acidity or alkalinity in your physiological state, thereby indicating the necessity of seeking a remedy to rectify this imbalance. If you are seeking means by which to assess your pH level, here are three approaches to initiate the testing process.

UNDERGO A BLOOD TEST

Arguably, the most effective approach to determine one's pH level involves conducting a blood sample examination under the guidance of a medical professional. The phlebologist subsequently performs a live cell microscopy procedure to ascertain the pH level of your system. The pH level of an individual's blood should ideally fall within the range of 7.35 to 7.45 to signify a state of good health. Any value that falls below or exceeds this range may potentially have a detrimental impact on your health.

Although opting for a blood test provides the utmost precision in ascertaining your pH levels, it entails considerable costs and demands significant investment of time. Therefore, it would not be the most optimal option if you intend to monitor your pH level over a specific duration.

Chapter 3:
Foods and Moods

Since my childhood, I have consistently encountered reactions to specific foods. Whenever I consumed pizza, cake, or ice cream, as illustrative examples, my emotional state would undergo a noticeable alteration. Soon after consuming my meal, my demeanor would undergo a transformation, transitioning from that of a contented child to that of a weeping young girl without discernible cause. This occurrence transpired consistently whenever I attended celebratory gatherings. I would experience an abrupt desire to return home and would proceed to contact my mother. Considering my mother's observational skills, she would inquire, "What was the fare consumed by you during the party?" Did you have pizza? When offered the choice between cake and ice cream, my lack of response would convey my preference.

The consumption of food exerts a significant impact on our emotional states. A significant number of individuals lack comprehension regarding the correlation and frequently undervalue the influence that food exerts over our emotional state and cognitive capabilities. Scientific research has demonstrated the impact of dietary choices on the neurochemicals responsible for cognitive function, memory consolidation, and emotional well-being.

A significant portion of the population experiences food intolerances and allergies. Certain individuals may exhibit a physiological response to food, resulting in manifestations such as the appearance of hives, swelling of the eyes and throat, and in severe cases, potentially fatal reactions to allergenic foods. Conversely, there are individuals who may experience subtler adverse reactions to foods they are intolerant to.

The bloodstream serves as a conduit for distributing the essential nutrients present in the consumed food to the entire body, including the brain. When we consume food, chemicals are released in both the intestinal and cerebral regions of our body. Certain chemical compounds have the propensity to induce heightened state of alertness, vitality, and well-being within our beings. Others elicit feelings of drowsiness or moodiness in us. The consumption of food that our bodies are intolerant to can elicit adverse physiological responses.

Acidic food items are frequently associated with the emergence of food allergies and intolerances, along with the consequent detrimental effects on physical well-being and mood disruptions. During my childhood, I lacked awareness regarding this matter, consequently consuming acidic foods that disrupted my Alkaline/Acid Balance.

As I reached adulthood, I acquired the understanding that modifying my dietary habits granted me the capacity to regulate my emotional states. After adopting an alkaline lifestyle, my life underwent a significant transformation. I was no longer afflicted with morning lethargy, rendering me unable on certain occasions to rise from bed. I ceased experiencing a lack of relaxation, and I ceased experiencing a sense of desolation. I discovered that I would eagerly spring out of bed each morning, prepared to embrace any new opportunities that would present themselves. I experienced a sense of rejuvenation, and my physical appearance exuded vitality and contentment.

I could not have authored this book in the past when I experienced profound fatigue and illness, coupled with pronounced fluctuations in temperament. I depended on the consumption of caffeine and sugary substances to sustain me throughout my daily activities. Furthermore, engaging in such actions left me with a sense of discomfort.

At present, I am able to sustain my energy levels without recourse to caffeine or the consumption of sugar. I am experiencing a profound sense of well-being, and I have ceased to encounter pronounced fluctuations in my mood throughout the course of the day. I am appreciative of the fact that I experienced feelings of discomfort, unwellness, and despondency. As I have gained awareness of the extent to which I can experience positive emotions in contrast. Through the experiences of adversity stemming from my personal health struggles, I have gained a profound understanding of the distinction between a state of imbalance and the attainment of optimal Alkaline/Acid Balance. Furthermore, I would not have been capable of disseminating this significant information to you.

I perceive the challenges I have encountered in the past as a fortuitous boon. As a result of the challenges I have faced, I have developed a profound belief in my own abilities. To ascertain the extent of my inner potential. To comprehend the extent of our collective potential. It has consistently remained in existence.

You possess the necessary qualities as well. Is today not the appropriate day to commence? Might this not be the opportune moment to reclaim your well-being and restore your emotional equilibrium, allowing you to revel in the joy and energy that you truly merit?

The Comprehensive Alkaline Diet Compendium

Alright, it seems that we have yet to cover what could arguably be considered the most crucial section of our book discussing the alkaline diet. This chapter will provide you with an overview of the permissible dietary options and those that should be avoided throughout the course of this nutritional regimen. Additionally, you will acquire the skills to effectively manage dining occasions with your companions while aligning them with your dietary goals. Moreover, you will gain insights on leveraging nutritional supplements to optimize your health and well-being. Ultimately, a comprehensive meal plan recommendation is provided to offer insights into the typical composition of a day adhering to the alkaline diet.

The PRAL Scale

Despite its lack of linguistic fluidity, the PRAL scale proves highly beneficial within the context of the alkaline diet.

The PRAL value signifies the degree of alkalinity or acidity found within a specific food. This implies that our approach involves evaluating the PRAL score of food items to determine the level and nature of their alkalinity or acidity, instead of merely categorizing them as either alkaline or acidic.

The PRAL metric assesses the pH balance of food by evaluating the residual protein, minerals, and phosphorus content following its metabolism within the human body. If the substance exhibits the presence of magnesium, calcium, and potassium residues, it is categorized as having an alkaline promoting effect, whereas the detection of phosphoric and sulfuric acid residues indicates its classification as acid forming. Taking into consideration the aforementioned point, let us now proceed to examine the dietary choices that are recommended and should be abstained from in adherence to an alkaline regimen.

Recommended Food Choices

In essence, vegetables and fruits, along with a variety of seeds and nuts, can be characterized as the predominant alkaline foods on the PRAL scale. Presented below is a compilation of nourishing food options that should be incorporated into your dietary regimen.

Beet Greens

Based on the PRAL scale, beet greens rank as the most alkaline food globally. Although they may not be widely renowned in our dietary practices, consider incorporating them into your stir-fries, smoothies, salads, or soups. They have the ability to substitute for any other green, however, caution is advised as they possess a slight bitter flavor. This attribute of bitterness, in fact, serves as a positive quality since it aids in stimulating the secretion of bile, thereby enhancing the digestion of fats.

Spinach

Spinach possesses a remarkable abundance of calcium, rendering it a highly favorable internal component that can significantly contribute to the enhancement of bone health.

Furthermore, it possesses a multitude of purifying juices that facilitate the detoxification of your body, consequently contributing to the potential prevention of cancer. Fortunately, there are numerous approaches to fostering creativity in the preparation of spinach, rendering it an ideal ingredient for incorporating into smoothies.

Kale

I am aware that individuals who prioritize meat consumption may express their disdain, however, kale has emerged as a formidable alternative to beef. It boasts high levels of calcium, iron, and vitamin K, rendering it beneficial for cancer prevention. In addition to this, its subtle flavor lends itself seamlessly to any culinary preparation. Regardless of whether you prefer it in a salad, stir-fry, or soup, the consumption of kale can provide a remarkable increase in alkalinity.

Swiss Chard

It is apparent that you have observed that our listings have predominantly consisted of leafy greens up until now. Indeed, it is correct that these foods hold the distinction of being the most alkaline in the world. Consequently, they should be regarded as the essential component of your revolutionary dietary approach.

With regards to Swiss chard, it possesses an abundance of vitamins, specifically vitamin K, which, as already mentioned, is of significant importance in the prevention of cancer. Furthermore, in addition to containing plant protein and phosphorus, it does not possess acidic properties. The basis for this lies in the fact that Swiss chard exhibits a significantly higher quantity of alkalizing minerals. Should you not have done so already, it is worth considering the substitution of Swiss chard in place of a tortilla in any given recipe.

Bananas

Bananas are renowned for their high fiber content, which plays a vital role in supporting optimal digestive function and purifying the gastrointestinal system. Indeed, bananas also contain a significant amount of fructose, a natural sugar found in fruits. Consequently, individuals concerned with their weight tend to refrain from consuming them. Nevertheless, bananas will perpetually remain a superior alternative in comparison to, for instance, a granola bar or any other food that encourages acidity.

Sweet Potatoes

Sweet potatoes possess notable alkaline properties, albeit their starch content necessitates moderate consumption. With a PRAL score indicating alkalinity, these foods possess the ability to augment your body's mineral, vitamin, and fiber intake. The high fiber content of these foods enables them to have minimal impact on blood sugar levels due to the gradual release of sugar into the bloodstream facilitated by fiber. This implies that sweet potatoes can provide a significant increase in energy levels, but it is important to consume them in moderation.

Celery

Celery plays a crucial role in the alkaline diet due to its purifying properties. The substantial water content aids in the rapid detoxification of our bodies. Furthermore, celery possesses immense value as an ingredient in any dietary regimen due to its negative calorie index. This implies that the energy expended during the process of chewing and digesting celery exceeds the caloric content contained within the celery itself.

Carrots

It is conceivable that during your early years, your parents may have advised you to consume carrots due to their potential benefits for vision improvement. Indeed, that statement holds true, for carrots possess a significant amount of vitamin A, which accounts for this phenomenon. Surprisingly, a mere cup of carrots contains a quantity of beta-carotene that exceeds three times the recommended daily amount, representing a significant intake of vitamin A. In addition to improving visual acuity, it also enhances dermatological well-being resulting in a more youthful appearance, besides potentially exerting a preventive influence on carcinogenesis.

Kiwi

Kiwi is an alternative dietary option that is abundant in essential minerals, vitamins, and antioxidants. Interestingly, oranges have gained widespread recognition for their high vitamin C content; however, it is worth noting that kiwi actually contains four times the amount of vitamin C. Furthermore, aside from its aforementioned benefits, the dietary fiber present in this substance aids in digestion, while the inclusion of potassium contributes to the optimal functioning of your muscular system.

Cauliflower

Females with elevated levels of estrogen should consider incorporating cauliflower into their diet as it may assist in restoring hormonal equilibrium. This outcome is attained via the utilization of Indole-3-Carbinol, an essential constituent that facilitates the regulation of estrogen levels within our physiological system. One may experience increased levels of estrogen as a result of consuming foods with estrogenic properties such as soy, using oral contraceptives, or being exposed to environmental chemicals such as plastics. Elevated estrogen levels can contribute to weight gain, induce bloating, and potentially result in infertility and the development of reproductive malignancies. Cauliflower can effectively contribute to the regulation of estrogen levels.

Cherries

Cherry is an additional inclusion to our inventory of alkaline promoting foods. They possess an abundance of antioxidants that can serve in safeguarding against the development of cancer. Furthermore, in addition to this, they are associated with the safeguarding of cardiovascular well-being and can contribute to alleviating the discomfort associated with arthritis and joint conditions. Cherries make a valuable inclusion to smoothies, while they can also be savored as a nutritious snack.

Eggplant

Eggplant introduces beneficial phytonutrients, including chlorogenic acid, into your system, promoting overall health. Notwithstanding its nomenclature as an acid, this compound possesses properties that effectively contribute to metabolic activities and facilitate the process of digestion due to its botanical origin. Eggplant serves as a superb complement to salads, and it can also be prepared through the process of baking within a conventional oven.

Pears

Pears belong to the category of fruits that possess low sugar content, rendering them a commendable option for individuals experiencing difficulties in maintaining balanced blood sugar levels. They also possess high levels of dietary fiber and vitamin C, both of which are pivotal in providing protection against the development of cancer.

Hazelnuts

Hazelnuts possess a unique quality among nuts as they exhibit an alkalizing impact. They serve as an excellent alternative to peanuts that have high acidity, making them the ideal snack option.

Pineapple

Contrary to popular belief, pineapple can indeed be found in certain nutritional supplements, serving as a testament to its beneficial impact on the human body. The underlying cause behind this phenomenon is the presence of bromelain, an enzymatic compound that actively eradicates intestinal parasites and enhances the process of digestion.

Zucchini

Zucchini is a crucial component of your alkaline diet due to the presence of lutein, an antioxidant belonging to the same category as beta-carotene. That indicates that it can contribute to maintaining unimpeded eyesight. Zucchini is additionally an essential component of diverse low-carbohydrate dietary plans, and it can serve as a superb substitute for pasta.

How Alkalinity Works

Welcome! We sincerely appreciate your acquisition of this book. Collectively, we shall delve into the possibilities presented by adhering to an alkaline diet, while also discussing its entrenched position in my personal existence. Furthermore, we will examine how you can incorporate this remarkable notion into your own life, leading to transformative health benefits with astounding celerity.

I have experimented with numerous dietary regimens in the past. In my opinion, emphasizing the augmentation of alkalinity is one of the most comprehensive approaches. This dietary plan inherently enhances the uptake of essential vitamins, nutrients, folic acid, and similar constituents. You will have the opportunity to consume a substantial amount of nutrient-rich vegetables, including peppers and other wholesome food choices. Nevertheless, you are partaking in the consumption of these foods with a novel objective: to heighten alkalinity levels, restore equilibrium to your body's pH, and attain the pinnacle of well-being.

As denoted by the title of this literary work, my objective is to facilitate a rapid improvement in your state of health. This is accomplished through a two-pronged approach encompassing the comprehensive transformation of your dietary habits, as well as the augmentation of your physical fitness regimen.

This book centers its attention on the previous. There exist numerous approaches to incorporate a new dietary regimen into your lifestyle, and alkalinity represents merely one tactic. Nevertheless, I highly recommend considering alkalinity, as there is a wealth of compelling research indicating the positive impact it can have on multiple facets of your physiological well-being.

Certain outcomes that have been documented as a result of adhering to this particular dietary plan encompass:

- There is a diminished risk of developing various diseases, including certain types of cancers.
- Obesity reduction - Decrease in body mass - Attainment of a healthier weight - Slimming down
- Enhanced emotional state - Heightened psychological well-being - Elevated mood - Augmented emotional outlook - Enhanced mental disposition
- Decreased inflammatory response
- Increased levels of energy

"Allow us to commence our investigation into the concept of alkalinity:

"The Importance of pH Levels

The term "pH" represents the acronym for potential hydrogen. The pH value of a solution represents its concentration of hydrogen ions. The pH reading will increase proportionally with the level of oxygen and alkalinity present in the fluid. As the pH reading decreases, the solution becomes increasingly acidic and depleted of oxygen. The pH scale spans a range of values extending from 0 to 14. The value of 7 represents a neutral state, with values higher than 7 indicating alkaline conditions and values lower than 7 indicating acidity.

Excessive alkalinity or acidity can both be toxic. It is imperative for the body/blood to maintain a state of neutrality or slight alkalinity, typically measured as 7.4 on the pH scale. Should the pH level significantly decrease below this threshold (resulting in acidity) or increase beyond acceptable limits (resulting in alkalinity), it indicates the presence of an underlying pathological condition. In the event of a significant shift in the chart, cellular death ensues, leading to the cessation of bodily functions ultimately resulting in mortality.

Of course, this is the pH levels of our functioning organs and bloodstream; but some parts of the body may vary greatly. For instance, the stomach harbors highly acidic conditions of significant potency. The oral cavity and saliva can undergo alterations towards acidic environments as a consequence of recently consumed food, or when confronted with a medical condition such as acid reflux.

Nevertheless, maintaining pH levels within the range of 7.4-7.5 is of utmost significance for the proper functioning of the remaining parts of your body. This represents your slightly alkaline reference point, and in the event that your body shifts towards acidic conditions, it can lead to several potential health implications.

Research by Gerry Schwalfenberg

In accordance with a scholarly article from 2011 authored by Dr. Schwalfenberg at the University of Alberta, the proven benefits of alkalinity have been established[1]. Schwalfenberg initiates his investigation by ascribing the declining pH levels observed worldwide to various ecological issues beyond the adverse impacts solely on human health.

The cause of this phenomenon can be attributed to the process of industrialization. As ecological disasters transpire, there is a corresponding correlation with acidity levels. The augmentation of carbon dioxide deposition has led to a modest rise in acidity levels in the Earth's oceans, which may have dire consequences, such as the potential devastation of coral reefs. Schwalfenberg highlights that the observation of reduced pH levels can help to identify a significant number of the global environmental issues. For example, in the event of a chemical leakage such as an oil spill in the ocean, it is probable that the acidity of the affected area will escalate. Consequently, this elevated acidity levels might lead to the demise of smaller organisms, thereby disrupting the delicate balance of the food chain and precipitating the extinction of certain species.

The subsequent matter to consider pertains to the pH levels of the human body, naturally. Essentially, our dietary composition has shifted towards a higher acidity level since the era of our hunter gatherer ancestors, commonly referred to as the paleolithic period. Ever since the advent of agriculture, we have pursued the refinement of grains into white breads. More recently, with the advent of food industrialization and the incorporation of various chemicals, preservatives, chlorides, and similar substances, our dietary habits have led to a significant increase in our overall acidity levels. Hence, this can be ascribed to numerous diseases that were not previously a concern in the past.

After thoroughly examining the literature on alkalinity, Schwalfenberg draws several conclusions:

- Enhanced alkalinity, achieved through an augmentation of the consumption of appropriate fruits and vegetables, is anticipated to positively impact various aspects such as bone health, mitigate muscle degeneration, alleviate the occurrence of chronic ailments like hypertension, and ultimately diminish the likelihood of strokes.

- Enhanced functionality of the endocrine system leads to an elevation in specific natural growth hormones. As a consequence, enhanced cardiovascular well-being, cognitive function, and memory are evident.

An alkaline diet has the capacity to elevate magnesium levels, thus facilitating the activation of vitamin D. This consequential enhancement of bodily functions and subsequent mitigation of diseases are observed.

Additionally, alkalinity has been found to provide support for individuals undergoing cancer treatment.

Ultimately, Schwalfenberg emphasizes the importance of utilizing appropriate soil for cultivating crops. An impoverished and acidic soil has the potential to yield produce that is of lesser quality compared to its healthy soil counterparts. Hence, it is advisable to endeavor to frequent farmer's markets and opt for locally cultivated produce whenever feasible. In the event that the pH level of soil falls into the range of 5, it is perceived as highly acidic, which may pose issues for the growth of your edible crops.

Schwalfenberg's research holds significance due to his diligent examination of numerous journals spanning the past few decades, all of which pertain to the correlation between health and alkalinity. There has been substantial discourse regarding the efficacy of alkalinity as a dietary approach, yet dismissing the significance of this regimen has become significantly more challenging.

In addition to Schwalfenberg's reportage, extensive research exists regarding the potential of elevated levels of alkalinity to diminish tumor growth, facilitate weight reduction, enhance metabolic functioning, augment energy levels, and mitigate free radical harm, consequently inducing anti-aging properties.

The Principle of the Alkaline Diet

In order to maintain optimal physical well-being and minimize the risk of illness, it is essential to incorporate a balanced dietary approach known as an alkaline or acid-alkaline diet. Essentially, it is a hypothesis positing that upon consumption of food, subsequent processes such as digestion and metabolism result in the generation of either an alkaline or acidic residue within the body, thereby determining its acid-alkaline balance.

The alkaline diet theory is predicated upon the contention that the pH level of our physiological systems is marginally basic, ranging from 7.35 to 7.45, as documented in certain scholarly texts, which alternatively state a range of 7.36 to 7.44. Our dietary intake should reflect this equilibrium. An alteration of this equilibrium will give rise to certain significant issues within the body. The acidity or alkalinity of a liquid is ascertained by the pH scale. It spans a scale from 0, indicating a highly acidic substance, to 14, representing an extremely alkaline substance. The pH of 7 corresponds to the neutral point, resembling that of water. A pH value that falls below 7 indicates acidity, which progressively strengthens as it descends. Conversely, a pH above 7 corresponds to alkaline substances, where the intensity amplifies as it ascends towards 14.

Almost all types of medical research possess underlying foundations in alkaline diets, albeit this theory remains unrecognized by conventional medical societies. In order to uphold the body's equilibrium, it is recommended to follow diets that consist of 60% alkaline substances. In order to restore equilibrium in the body, individuals should incorporate predominantly alkaline diets, accounting for 80% of their food intake, as the excessive consumption of meat, eggs, cream, and other acidic foods has disrupted the balance.

When considering alkaline diets, it is advisable to prioritize the consumption of vegetables, low-fat fruits, nuts, tubers, fresh citrus, and similar items. To enhance the alkalinity in the body, one can utilize fruits as a viable source, given that fruits generally contain substantial amounts of alkaline compounds. Only a limited quantity of fruits exhibit acidic properties. When consuming fruits for this objective, it is advisable to abstain from consuming canned, sugared, or preserved variants, as they undergo significant acidity alteration during the preservation process owing to the incorporation of various chemical compounds.

Within the context of alkaline diet principles, vegetables come highly endorsed due to their substantial capacity to promote an alkaline state within the body. If the meat you consume undergoes acidification in your body, conventional doctors, who may not acknowledge the potential benefits of vegetable consumption, advocate for the consumption of meat in order to derive energy. Consequently, you are likely to experience a sense of weakness rather than empowerment in your physical being.

Vegetables, particularly those of the green variety, serve as excellent sources of alkaline production. They can be utilized not only in cooked form but also in their raw state. Vegetables such as carrots, cauliflower, tomatoes, and various others can be consumed at any time without the need for cooking. They possess a delectable flavor while offering an abundance of essential minerals. Mineral elements such as calcium, potassium, and magnesium serve as the primary contributors to alkaline ash, and they play a vital role in promoting the growth and proper functioning of the human body. Our body undergoes a transformation from an acidic state to a mildly alkaline state as a result of the reaction between these minerals and the acid existing within our body.

Chapter 2. Guidelines for Properly Adhering to the Alkaline Diet

Enhancement of Health Conditions Through the Adoption of an Alkaline Diet

The efficacy of the alkaline diet has been substantiated in the treatment of the subsequent health conditions:

Arthritis
Diabetes
Cancer
Insomnia
Muscle Pain
Gout
Bloating

Alkaline Water?

Typically, water exhibits a pH level of 7, known as the state of neutrality. Alkaline water typically possesses an elevated pH level, usually ranging from 8 to 9. This water assists in preserving the alkaline state of the gastrointestinal tract. It is employed as a means to facilitate detoxification and provide treatment, elicits anti-aging benefits, and possesses the potential to combat cancer and obesity.

Common Inquiries Regarding the Alkaline Diet

Q. What is the correlation between alkaline food consumption and the occurrence of acid reflux?
Acid reflux is a condition characterized by a sensation of intense heat or burning within the stomach, stemming from an excessive secretion of hydrochloric acid in the gastric region. Alkaline food is intentionally employed for the treatment of acid reflux, as it inhibits the consumption of food that promotes acid formation.

Q. How alkaline food can treat obesity?
The alkaline diet offers a strategic approach for weight reduction and obesity treatment by eliminating sugars, complex carbohydrates, and saturated fats.

Q. Does the act of cooking cause alkaline food to become acidic?

I'm sorry, but that assertion is entirely inaccurate. Cooking alkaline food does not lead to its acidification. Nevertheless, the inclusion of an acidic component in the dish leads to an overall acidity.

Nutritional Classification: Alkaline and Acidic Food Groups

Food that has the ability to lower the acidity of the gastrointestinal system is referred to as acid-forming food, while food items that increase the internal pH level are known as alkaline-forming food.

Acid-Forming Foods

Enclosed herewith is the comprehensive inventory of food items that have an acidic effect:

Rice options available: white, brown, or basmati.

All types of meat are available, including beef, pork, lamb, fish, and chicken.

Popcorn
Cornmeal, rye
Colas
Cheese
Pasta
Wheat germ
Alcoholic drinks
Coffee and other beverages containing caffeine
Soy sauce
Sweetened yogurt
Mustard
Ketchup
Refined table salt
Mayonnaise
White vinegar
Nutmeg
Tobacco

Alkalinizing Foods
"Please find enclosed an exhaustive catalogue of alkaline food items:
Varieties of beans such as string, soy, lima, green, and snap
Peas
Potatoes
Arrowroot flour

Examples of cereals include flax, millet, quinoa, and amaranth.

Nuts such as almonds, freshly harvested coconuts, and chestnuts.

Germinated seeds of alfalfa, radish, and chia "

Unsprouted sesame

Fresh unsalted butter

Whey

Plain yogurt

Fruit juices

All vegetable juices

Most herbal teas

Garlic

Cayenne pepper

Gelatin

Most herbs

Miso

The majority of vegetables and unrefined sea salt.

Most all spices

Vanilla extract

Natural sweeteners such as unprocessed, non-pasteurized honey, dehydrated sugar cane juice (Sucanat), and brown rice syrup

Brewer's yeast

Chapter 1 our health

If you have taken basic biology lesson, you will know that cells require certain conditions to function normally. Accurate manipulation of temperature and pH is imperative to facilitate the sustenance of basic life forms. The human body, despite its apparent durability and exemption from this principle, is actually no exception. It requires basic conditions in order to have optimal performance.

When the human body is operating at its peak efficiency, bodily fluids and tissues maintain a slightly alkaline condition, rather than an acidic one. The nourishment ingested frequently serves as the fundamental substance required for the regeneration of bodily tissues. Our body's pH levels can easily become imbalanced if a significant portion of our diet comprises foods that have an acidifying effect.

The dietary patterns adhered to by our predecessors starkly contrast with the familiar customs we presently embrace.

As technology progresses, there is a ripple effect on the variety of foods we incorporate into our diets. A visit to the supermarket will astound you with its vast array of processed food items and animal-derived products. Locating fast food establishments while dining out will not pose any difficulty, as they are readily available on nearly every street corner.

Fad diets, to some extent, also bear responsibility for the introduction of novel dietary practices, such as the adoption of high-protein regimens. In recent years, there has been a surge in the consumption of animal products and refined food items, as an increasing number of individuals have omitted the inclusion of daily servings of fruits and vegetables in their dietary regimen. It is not surprising that in contemporary times, numerous individuals are experiencing diverse allergic conditions, ailments affecting the bones, cardiovascular issues, and various other health problems. Several health professionals attribute these diseases to the dietary choices we make. Certain categories of food have the potential to disturb a specific equilibrium within our body, thereby giving rise to various health complications. If only we could alter our dietary practices, it is not implausible that we may attain disease prevention and the restoration of health. The human body possesses several organ systems which are proficient at counteracting and expelling surplus acid, yet there exists a threshold beyond which even a robust physique can no longer efficiently manage an excessive acid load. The human body possesses the ability to sustain an appropriate acid-alkaline equilibrium, on the condition that the bodily organs are in proper working order and an adequately balanced alkaline diet is being ingested.

What methods can be employed to determine the pH level of one's body?

and requires your attention? Below is a prescribed course of action to determine whether your body is excessively acidic. It is advised to commence by introspectively assessing if any of the symptoms listed herein are prevalent in your experience.

a. Pimples & Acnes b. Agitation c. Rapid panting breath d. Rapid heartbeat e. Muscular pain f. Pain experienced before and during menstruation. Pre-menstrual anxiety and depression are common occurrences among women during the pre-menstrual phase. I am experiencing sensations of coldness in my hands and feet. Syncope and vertigo. Prone to fatigue and experiencing diminished vitality. Articular discomfort that migrates. Food allergies m. Excessive gas n. Hyperactivity o. Diminished libido. Bloating q. Gastroesophageal reflux disease (GERD). Urine that is yellow in color and emits a strong odor. Headaches & migraines t. Irregular heartbeat u. White coated tongue v. It is challenging to awaken in the morning.

Excessive nasal congestion: If you exhibit more than two of the symptoms described above, it is highly probable that your body is experiencing acidity, and it is advisable to exercise caution and modify your dietary habits in order to prevent the accumulation of toxins that could potentially lead to serious ailments, including cancer, over time. The fact remains that a significant portion of individuals have been consuming food incorrectly. The concept of a "balanced" diet, which educated us about food pyramids, well-rounded meals, and nutritious foods, is responsible for our increasing rates of obesity, disease, and poor health. And this is due to the fact that a diet that is skewed towards meat, dairy, and grains results in an acidic composition of meals. Do you frequently experience fatigue, particularly after consuming a meal? In reality, this tiredness often occurs around the hours of 3-4 pm (subject to the time at which you have lunch), when you encounter challenges in maintaining wakefulness. You experience pronounced fatigue, extreme weariness, and an inability to sustain your work efforts. In light of recent research, it has come to my attention that an intriguing explanation exists for our current experience. The underlying cause for

153

this sensation can be attributed to the excessive energy required by our bodies to undertake the process of digesting our midday meal. Between the hours of 3 and 4 pm, our bodily systems have already undergone significant exertion for a substantial portion of the day. In light of the energy expenditure required for digestion following our midday meal, it is inherent for our body to instinctively seek a period of repose. In the past, I held the belief that this occurrence is innate - it is only natural to experience lethargy during the afternoon...

However, my initial assumption proved to be mistaken.

The reality is that the manner in which we consume our meals, as well as the types of food we ingest, have deleterious implications for our physical well-being and overall health. As an illustration, do you partake in the consumption of meat and potatoes in conjunction with one another? Might I suggest pairing milk and cereal, or perhaps fish and rice? Are you aware that those combinations have a profoundly detrimental impact on your internal system, depleting your energy reserves?

One may perceive this as absurd..

Allow me to elucidate the detrimental nature of these combinations and present to you an opportunity to conserve significant amounts of energy that you may presently be squandering. Various types of food undergo distinct digestive processes - Alimentary items rich in starch necessitate an alkaline environment for digestion, whereas protein-rich foods such as meat call for an acidic medium. When the combination of both entities occurs, the medium subsequently undergoes a process of neutralization. Digestive function is compromised or completely halted. This has a highly negative impact on your physical health, as it necessitates a greater expenditure of energy to effectively metabolize the same quantity of food. Did you experience a similar level of astonishment as I did when you were first made aware of this? What course of action can be taken to address this matter? The initial lesson I acquired was that of consuming appropriate food choices and refraining from combining incompatible food items. As an illustration, in the event that I consume starchy foods, I would refrain from including meat within the same meal. If I were consuming meat, I would refrain from incorporating starchy foods. If you are contemplating the efficacy of this approach, I would encourage you to attempt it and observe any discernible physiological changes. I have personally experimented with this dietary approach, which not only allows for the consumption of a wide range of foods but also greatly enhances one's overall state of health.

Fundamental Tenets of the Alkaline Dietary Regimen
The alkaline diet comprises a substantial amount of nutrients and fiber, alongside beneficial fats rich in anti-inflammatory omega-3s. It is deficient in animal-sourced proteins and processed dietary

items. On the whole, the majority of these fundamental principles contribute to mitigating the potential of developing diseases such as cancer.

The foundation of a nutritious alkaline diet regimen rests upon five fundamental steps. Presented below, these recommendations can provide guidance in adjusting your dietary habits and food selections in alignment with a high alkaline diet, ultimately promoting improved overall health.

1. Seek out fresh, unprocessed food alternatives, with a preference for organic produce. Adopting a dietary approach that revolves around whole foods and limiting consumption of trans fats, processed sugar, and heavily refined products forms the fundamental cornerstone of any endeavor toward a health-conscious lifestyle. The alkaline diet is based on this fundamental principle. In addition, vegetables should be prepared raw or lightly steamed. Cooking or frying vegetables is not advisable as it can lead to the depletion of nutrients.

2. Consume a diverse range of food items: Consuming a diverse range of food items, with an emphasis on foods that align with an alkaline diet, can contribute to the promotion of a healthy digestive system and the efficient functioning of bodily processes. Adopting an alkaline diet regimen that incorporates a higher proportion of plant-based ingredients and dietary fiber has been scientifically substantiated to diminish the likelihood of developing cancer and various other persistent ailments. Commence perusing newly available seasonal produce at your nearby farmer's market - this can enhance the enjoyment of meal planning and promote a healthier eating regimen.

3. Ensure adequate consumption of water: Maintaining proper hydration is a crucial aspect of any dietary regimen, including the alkaline diet. Ensuring adequate hydration, preferably through the consumption of filtered water, can support your body in effectively digesting dietary modifications and an elevated intake of dietary fiber. This will

aid in the elimination and reduction of deleterious waste substances from your body.

4. Refrain from consuming foods to which you have allergies, as their ingestion can incite inflammation, irrespective of the overall alkalinity or acidity of the food. Identify and avoid those food allergies.

5. Give priority to alkaline foods: Depending on your specific requirements, it is advisable to include a combination of both alkaline and acidic foods in your diet. Nevertheless, the prioritization of alkaline foods will ensure that your overall dietary choices are conducive to reducing inflammation, minimizing food reactions, and promoting optimal detoxification processes. Adopting a practice of reducing and restricting the consumption of acidic foods, which have been linked to elevated risks of cancer, is an excellent initial measure towards enhancing one's overall well-being.

www.ingramcontent.com/pod-product-compliance
Lightning Source LLC
Chambersburg PA
CBHW051734020426
42333CB00014B/1309